COUNTDOWN TO MY BIRTH

A day-by-day account from your baby's point of view

Julie Carr

 **Meadowbrook Press**
Distributed by Simon & Schuster
New York

Library of Congress Control Number: 2014953558

Editors: Angela Wiechmann, Megan McGinnis
Production Manager: Paul Woods
Creative Director: Tamara JM Peterson
Cover Photography: Olesia Bilkei

Published by:
Meadowbrook Press
6110 Blue Circle Drive Suite 237
Minnetonka, Minnesota 55343

www.MeadowbrookPress.com

BOOK TRADE DISTRIBUTION by:
Simon and Schuster
a division of Simon and Schuster, Inc.
1230 Avenue of the Americas
New York, NY 10020

20 19 18 17 16 15 14   10 9 8 7 6 5 4 3 2 1

Printed in USA

Acknowledgements

This book is dedicated to Dave
and my own little miracles,
PJ and Benjamin, with love.

Special thanks to Rachel Bye, MD,
for her thorough medical
review of the contents.

Disclaimer

All women and pregnancies are unique, and all babies develop at different rates. The information in *Countdown to My Birth* represents estimated progress during pregnancy and may not correspond to exact developments on a daily basis. Weights and lengths are estimates and will vary from baby to baby.

This book is not intended to be a substitute for the medical advice of a trained health care professional or a replacement for your regularly scheduled prenatal appointments. Please consult your health care provider for any questions or concerns you may have.

Instructions

The Weeks and Days of Pregnancy

This calendar is based on a 40-week pregnancy, starting with the first day of your last menstrual period (LMP). Keep in mind, however, your baby's *fetal age* will always be two weeks less than his or her *gestational age*, since conception occurs about two weeks after the first day of your LMP.

Please note the calendar counts the *completed* weeks and days of your pregnancy rather than the week or day of pregnancy you're *in*. On the first day of your LMP, you've completed "0 weeks, 0 days" of your pregnancy. You don't complete "1 day" until 24 hours have passed, and you don't complete "1 week" until seven days have passed.

Likewise, you've completed "2 weeks, 0 days" on the day you most likely conceive. Going forward, you've completed "2 weeks, 1 day," "2 weeks, 2 days," and so on until all seven days have passed, at which time you've completed "3 weeks, 0 days."

If you find this method hard to comprehend, compare it to how you'll soon keep track of your baby's age: Your baby will be *in* his or her first week from the moment of birth, but he or she isn't "1 week" old until all seven days have passed.

Filling in Your Dates

On the first calendar page, go to the first day's entry, "0 weeks, 0 days," write the date of the first day of your LMP in the "Today is" space provided at the bottom left corner. Then go to the next entry, "2 weeks, 0 days," and fill in the appropriate date for two weeks after the first day of your LMP, which is when you most likely conceived. (I don't include entries between the first day of your LMP and conception.)

Using a dated calendar as a guide, fill in each date for the next 40 weeks. Fill in your estimated due date at "40 weeks, 0 days." From there, fill in the dates for two additional weeks, since your baby likely won't arrive exactly on your due date. Alternate method: If you don't know the first day of your LMP, work backward from your estimated due date.

Be sure to use the Notes section on every page to write in appointments or journal your thoughts.

The Countdown

Although the title of this calendar is *Countdown to My Birth*, it's important to remember that unless you're having a scheduled cesarean section, you don't know exactly when that joyous event will occur! What you do know is your estimated due date, and you can guess your baby will likely be born anytime from two weeks before to two weeks after that date.

Therefore, in the bottom right corner of every entry is the countdown for "Days to due date." When you're "0 weeks, 0 days" pregnant, you have 280 days until your due date. When you're "0 weeks, 1 day" pregnant, you have 279 days to your due date, and so on. If your due date goes by and the baby still hasn't arrived, the countdown will keep track of "Days past due date." If you find yourself in that situation, rest assured that you're *not* "overdue" until two weeks past your due date.

I hope you and your new miracle enjoy *Countdown to My Birth* during this incredible time of discovery, and for years to come.

Sincerely,
Julie Carr

About the Author

Julie B. Carr is the president of Motherly Way Enterprises, Inc., and owner of the online pregnancy store MotherlyWay.com. She graduated from Westfield State College in Massachusetts with a degree in business management. After working in the computer industry for ten years, Julie left the high-tech world when she became a mother. Inspired during her pregnancy with her first son, she researched, wrote, and published the first edition of what was to become *Countdown to My Birth*. Julie lives in Oregon with her husband, Dave, and their two sons.

COUNTDOWN TO MY BIRTH

A day-by-day account from your baby's point of view

Get ready, Mom! You're not pregnant yet, but today is the first day of your last menstrual period (LMP). Your pregnancy will last approximately 40 weeks or 280 days starting today.

Notes:

Today is   /   /   **0** weeks, **0** days   Days to due date: **280**

Two weeks have passed, and today your ovary released an egg, and Dad's sperm fertilized it. Hurray! This is the beginning of the making of me!

Notes:

Today is   /   /   **2** weeks, **0** days   Days to due date: **266**

Chromosomes containing genetic material from both you and Dad fuse inside the egg. This magical moment determines whether I'll be a boy or a girl, what color my hair and eyes will be, and many other characteristics.

Notes:

Today is   /   /   **2** weeks, **1** days   Days to due date: **265**

COUNTDOWN TO MY BIRTH
A day-by-day account from your baby's point of view

Notes: _____

It's been 24 hours since your chromosomes fused, and now my single cell has divided into two. When another 18 hours have passed, I'll begin my three-day journey through your fallopian tube to my next destination: your uterus.

Today is ___ / ___ / ___   **2** weeks, **2** days   Days to due date: **264**

Notes: _____

As I travel through the fallopian tube, my cells divide into two sections. Some will become me; the rest will become the placenta to nourish me for the next nine months.

Today is ___ / ___ / ___   **2** weeks, **3** days   Days to due date: **263**

Notes: _____

Finally, after three days of traveling, I've reached your uterus—my new home for the next nine months. It'll take me a day or two to decide exactly where I'd like to attach.

Today is ___ / ___ / ___   **2** weeks, **4** days   Days to due date: **262**

COUNTDOWN TO MY BIRTH

A day-by-day account from your baby's point of view

Notes: _____

A fter checking out some different sites, I've picked a spot where I can attach to your uterus—most likely a place at the top.

Today is ___/___/___   **2 weeks, 5** days   Days to due date: **261**

Notes: _____

N ow that I'm settled in, the real work begins! I start by exchanging all sorts of chemicals and hormones with your body to let you know you're pregnant.

Today is ___/___/___   **2 weeks, 6** days   Days to due date: **260**

Notes: _____

I 'm growing steadily by dividing my cells again and again. I've grown from one cell to over 200 by now, and each cell looks totally different from the rest.

Today is ___/___/___   **3 weeks, 0** days   Days to due date: **259**

Notes:

I'm sending you more hormones and proteins so your body knows I'm not just some "foreign cells" hanging around!

Today is   /   /   **3** weeks, **1** days   Days to due date: **258**

Notes:

Although I'm incredibly small, I have the power to make you queasy from all the hormones I'm sending you—even at this early stage.

Today is   /   /   **3** weeks, **2** days   Days to due date: **257**

Notes:

My cells divide about twice a day. I now have several thousands of them.

Today is   /   /   **3** weeks, **3** days   Days to due date: **256**

Notes:

I'm still very tiny—only 0.04 inch (1 millimeter) long, which is the size of a grain of sugar.

Today is   /   /   **3** weeks, **4** days   Days to due date: **255**

Notes:

The next five weeks are very important—my heart and central nervous system are starting to form. Continuing to take your prenatal vitamin every day helps me do this complicated task.

Today is   /   /   **3** weeks, **5** days   Days to due date: **254**

Notes:

All my thousands of cells came from the original one at conception. One of the greatest mysteries is how different cells become different parts of me!

Today is   /   /   **3** weeks, **6** days   Days to due date: **253**

COUNTDOWN TO MY BIRTH
A day-by-day account from your baby's point of view

My cells are arranging into three separate layers—like a layered nacho dip. The outer layer will become my brain, nerves, and skin.

Notes:

Today is ___/___/___   **4** weeks, **0** days   Days to due date: **252**

The middle layer of this "nacho dip" will become the deeper layers of my skin as well as my bones, muscles, heart, reproductive organs, and blood vessels.

Notes:

Today is ___/___/___   **4** weeks, **1** days   Days to due date: **251**

The inner layer of these cells will become my intestines, lungs, and urinary tract. So many parts to form!

Notes:

Today is ___/___/___   **4** weeks, **2** days   Days to due date: **250**

COUNTDOWN TO MY BIRTH
A day-by-day account from your baby's point of view

Notes: _____

I feel a bump in my throat—my thyroid gland must be forming. This will help regulate my metabolism when I'm older.

Today is ___ / ___ / ___   **4 weeks, 3 days**   Days to due date: **249**

Notes: _____

I'm floating inside the amniotic sac, which will be my "house" for the next eight months. It's about the size of a grape now, but thankfully it'll expand as I grow!

Today is ___ / ___ / ___   **4 weeks, 4 days**   Days to due date: **248**

Notes: _____

Wow! I've doubled in size in the last nine days and am now 0.08 inch (2 millimeters) long.

Today is ___ / ___ / ___   **4 weeks, 5 days**   Days to due date: **247**

Notes: _____

If you could look at me right now, you'd see the beginning of my brain and backbone. Don't laugh, but I also have a little tail.

Today is ___/___/___   **4** weeks, **6** days   Days to due date: **246**

Notes: _____

Now my heart begins to beat and pump blood. Hurray! This is my first organ to function!

Today is ___/___/___   **5** weeks, **0** days   Days to due date: **245**

Notes: _____

My body is so small, my digestive system is starting to form inside my yolk sac. That's the membrane where I get nourishment, where my early blood is produced, and where some of my "pieces" develop when I need extra room.

Today is ___/___/___   **5** weeks, **1** days   Days to due date: **244**

Notes: _____

My body develops from the top and works its way down. Now my chin, cheeks, upper jaw, and ears or forming. You'll see my tiny face soon enough.

Today is   /   /   **5** weeks, **2** days   Days to due date: **243**

Notes: _____

My arms are starting to form. They look like little bumps on my body!

Today is   /   /   **5** weeks, **3** days   Days to due date: **242**

Notes: _____

I'm now about ¼ inch (6 millimeters) long—about the size of a pea. That's 10,000 times bigger than at conception!

Today is   /   /   **5** weeks, **4** days   Days to due date: **241**

Notes: _____

My legs are just beginning to form. They're developing a little more slowly than my arms, but soon enough, I'll be running circles around you!

Today is ___ / ___ / ___   5 weeks, 5 days   Days to due date: **240**

Notes: _____

Now my tiny liver, gallbladder, stomach, and lungs are beginning to develop.

Today is ___ / ___ / ___   5 weeks, 6 days   Days to due date: **239**

Notes: _____

Strange as it may seem, my heart is located on the outside of my body. It pumps about 85 times a minute.

Today is ___ / ___ / ___   6 weeks, 0 days   Days to due date: **238**

Notes: _____

Dark spots beneath my skin mark where my eyes and ears will appear. I can't wait to see your face and hear your voice after I'm born.

Today is ___ / ___ / ___   **6 weeks, 1** days   Days to due date: **237**

Notes: _____

My head had been bent way forward, but now I'm beginning to straighten my neck as well as the rest of my body. It's never too early to have good posture!

Today is ___ / ___ / ___   **6 weeks, 2** days   Days to due date: **236**

Notes: _____

Don't worry too much about any minor bumps and falls. My amniotic sac is filled with fluid, and I'm well protected as I float around.

Today is ___ / ___ / ___   **6 weeks, 3** days   Days to due date: **235**

Notes: _____

My neural tube closes over my spinal canal, and my nervous system begins to develop. This will become my body's "mission control center."

Today is ___/___/___   **6** weeks, **4** days   Days to due date: **234**

Notes: _____

I'm growing so fast. Since last week, I've almost doubled in length to ½ inch (13 millimeters) and will grow almost a millimeter a day. I weigh 0.00004 ounce (1 milligram). That's about as heavy as a small eyelash!

Today is ___/___/___   **6** weeks, **5** days   Days to due date: **233**

Notes: _____

My head and brain are growing rapidly—my head is almost as large as the rest of my body. Imagine if your head extended all the way to your hips!

Today is ___/___/___   **6** weeks, **6** days   Days to due date: **232**

Notes: _____

Different cells are still becoming different parts of me. Right now there are 12 rows of cells forming across my body. These will eventually become my ribs.

Today is ___/___/___ **7 weeks, 0** days Days to due date: **231**

Notes: _____

Here's looking at you, Mom! The lenses for my eyes are forming.

Today is ___/___/___ **7 weeks, 1** days Days to due date: **230**

Notes: _____

Even though my sex was determined at conception, my ovaries or testes are just starting to develop.

Today is ___/___/___ **7 weeks, 2** days Days to due date: **229**

Notes: _____

My arms had been straight, but now my elbows are forming. That should give me a little more "elbow room" in here!

Today is [/   /   ]   **7** weeks, **3** days   Days to due date: **228**

Notes: _____

My body is pretty rubbery. My whole skeleton is made of cartilage—just like the tip of your nose.

Today is [/   /   ]   **7** weeks, **4** days   Days to due date: **227**

Notes: _____

My skin is so thin it's transparent, as if I were wrapped in tissue paper. You can look through it and see my spinal column developing.

Today is [/   /   ]   **7** weeks, **5** days   Days to due date: **226**

Notes: _____

Does anyone have a lollipop? My tongue is now formed.

Today is ___/___/___   **7** weeks, **6** days   Days to due date: **225**

Notes: _____

No more wearing my heart on my sleeve! My heart has moved from the outside to the inside of my body, where it belongs.

Today is ___/___/___   **8** weeks, **0** days   Days to due date: **224**

Notes: _____

My arms are each as long as this exclamation point!

Today is ___/___/___   **8** weeks, **1** days   Days to due date: **223**

Notes: _____

Thanks for sending me oxygen through the umbilical cord, but eventually I'll need to breathe on my own. Little bumps that will become my lungs are now beginning to appear.

Today is ___/___/___   **8** weeks, **2** days   Days to due date: **222**

Notes: _____

I've reached a milestone: True bone cells begin to replace my cartilage, signaling my transition from an "embryo" to a "fetus."

Today is ___/___/___   **8** weeks, **3** days   Days to due date: **221**

Notes: _____

My hands and feet are partially formed and look like paddles. You can even make out my big toes!

Today is ___/___/___   **8** weeks, **4** days   Days to due date: **220**

Notes: _____

I'm now about 1 inch (25 millimeters) long—about the length of your fingerprint.

Today is ___ / ___ / ___   **8** weeks, **5** days   Days to due date: **219**

Notes: _____

At this tender age, all of my organs have already formed. Now my body needs to work on the details—and grow!

Today is ___ / ___ / ___   **8** weeks, **6** days   Days to due date: **218**

Notes: _____

I need lots of calcium now to make my teeth and bones, so help me out and eat plenty of dairy products and leafy green vegetables.

Today is ___ / ___ / ___   **9** weeks, **0** days   Days to due date: **217**

Notes: _____

I may be little, but I'm very active. I'm constantly moving around, although you won't feel me for another 7–15 weeks.

Today is ___/___/___   **9** weeks, **1** days   Days to due date: **216**

Notes: _____

The bones in my cheeks and chin are growing and fusing to eventually create my beautiful face.

Today is ___/___/___   **9** weeks, **2** days   Days to due date: **215**

Notes: _____

My eyes used to be on the sides of my head. Now they're moving toward the front so I'll look a little less "alien."

Today is ___/___/___   **9** weeks, **3** days   Days to due date: **214**

Notes:

Whether I'm a little boy or girl, my reproductive organs are now taking shape so I can create little "miracles" of my own in the future.

Today is ___ / ___ / ___   **9** weeks, **4** days   Days to due date: **213**

Notes:

I'm now about 1⅓ inches (3½ centimeters) long, which is the length of a small paper clip. I also weigh ⅛ ounce (4 grams). That's the weight of two sheets of paper.

Today is ___ / ___ / ___   **9** weeks, **5** days   Days to due date: **212**

Notes:

It was nice having extra help, but since my liver and spleen now produce my blood cells, I no longer need the yolk sac. It'll soon detach from me.

Today is ___ / ___ / ___   **9** weeks, **6** days   Days to due date: **211**

COUNTDOWN TO MY BIRTH

A day-by-day account from your baby's point of view

Notes: _____

Next time you do your nails, keep in mind that nail beds are beginning to form for my finger- and toenails.

Today is ___/___/___   **10** weeks, **0** days   Days to due date: **210**

Notes: _____

No more tadpole jokes—my tail is disappearing.

Today is ___/___/___   **10** weeks, **1** days   Days to due date: **209**

Notes: _____

M'm! *M'm*! Good! My taste buds are appearing on my tongue.

Today is ___/___/___   **10** weeks, **2** days   Days to due date: **208**

Notes: _____
_____
_____
_____

I now have 20 little buds for my baby teeth. If only teething later on were this easy!

Today is ___/___/___   **10** weeks, **3** days   Days to due date: **207**

Notes: _____
_____
_____
_____

My kidneys are still forming. You know what they say: "No guts, no glory!"

Today is ___/___/___   **10** weeks, **4** days   Days to due date: **206**

Notes: _____
_____
_____
_____

My heart is forming its four chambers. You can see them if you have an ultrasound.

Today is ___/___/___   **10** weeks, **5** days   Days to due date: **205**

Notes: _____

I want to keep my food in my mouth when I'm older, so my palate—the roof of my mouth—is closing.

Today is ___ / ___ / ___   **10** weeks, **6** days   Days to due date: **204**

Notes: _____

Don't expect any late-night conversations yet, but my vocal cords are complete.

Today is ___ / ___ / ___   **11** weeks, **0** days   Days to due date: **203**

Notes: _____

My heart beats 120–160 times per minute—twice as fast as yours.

Today is ___ / ___ / ___   **11** weeks, **1** days   Days to due date: **202**

Notes: _____

The placenta will weigh about 1½ pounds (908 grams) when I'm born. Right now, it weighs only about 1 ounce (28 grams), but it's bigger than I am!

Today is ___ / ___ / ___   **11** weeks, **2** days   Days to due date: **201**

Notes: _____

My heartbeat is getting stronger now. You can probably hear it at your prenatal checkup.

Today is ___ / ___ / ___   **11** weeks, **3** days   Days to due date: **200**

Notes: _____

Say it again, Sam! My ears are starting to form, but they won't be complete until the fifth month.

Today is ___ / ___ / ___   **11** weeks, **4** days   Days to due date: **199**

Notes: _____

I'm now about 3½ inches (9 centimeters) long, slightly longer than a credit card. I weigh about ½ ounce (14 grams), as much as a Magic Marker.

Today is ___/___/___   **11** weeks, **5** days   Days to due date: **198**

Notes: _____

My brain sends my muscles signals to kick and move. Unfortunately, my brain isn't organized enough yet to manage them, so I'm a little out of control.

Today is ___/___/___   **11** weeks, **6** days   Days to due date: **197**

Notes: _____

My intestines actually developed in my umbilical cord. I'm happy to say they're now moving into my body, where they belong.

Today is ___/___/___   **12** weeks, **0** days   Days to due date: **196**

Notes: _____

I can curl my toes, bend my arms at the elbows, flex my hands at the wrists, and form tight fists—what fun!

Today is ___ / ___ / ___   **12** weeks, **1** days   Days to due date: **195**

Notes: _____

My baby-teeth buds already formed two weeks ago, but now 32 buds for my permanent teeth appear. I'll have pearly whites to flash for photos when I'm older.

Today is ___ / ___ / ___   **12** weeks, **2** days   Days to due date: **194**

Notes: _____

Will I have Dad's hairline or yours? My scalp hair pattern will soon emerge as fuzzy white hair begins to form on my head.

Today is ___ / ___ / ___   **12** weeks, **3** days   Days to due date: **193**

Notes: _____

My head is still very large compared to the rest of me. Can you believe it's about one-third of my entire body length?

Today is ___/___/___   12 weeks, 4 days   Days to due date: **192**

Notes: _____

Think of all the body parts I already have, and yet I weigh only about 1 ounce (28 grams). That's as much as a slice of cheese!

Today is ___/___/___   12 weeks, 5 days   Days to due date: **191**

Notes: _____

Congratulations! We've now completed our first trimester!

Today is ___/___/___   12 weeks, 6 days   Days to due date: **190**

Notes: _____
_____
_____
_____
_____

I'm growing rapidly now.
During the next four weeks,
I'll grow approximately 2–3
more inches (5–8 centimeters).

_____
_____
_____
_____
_____

Today is ___ / ___ / ___   **13** weeks, **0** days   Days to due date: **189**

Notes: _____
_____
_____
_____

I'm looking more like a
baby now that my nostrils,
cheeks, lips, and chin are
better defined.

_____
_____
_____
_____
_____

Today is ___ / ___ / ___   **13** weeks, **1** days   Days to due date: **188**

Notes: _____
_____
_____
_____

As muscles attach to
my face, I can open
and close my mouth as
well as smile and frown.

_____
_____
_____
_____

Today is ___ / ___ / ___   **13** weeks, **2** days   Days to due date: **187**

Notes: _____

I'm developing some reflexes. If you could touch my palms, my fingers would close. Touching the inner soles of my feet would make my toes curl.

Today is ___ / ___ / ___   **13** weeks, **3** days   Days to due date: **186**

Notes: _____

My parts are still moving to the right places. My ears have now moved from my upper neck to my head.

Today is ___ / ___ / ___   **13** weeks, **4** days   Days to due date: **185**

Notes: _____

I'm getting pretty tall! I'm 5 inches (13 centimeters) or about as long as a taco shell.

Today is ___ / ___ / ___   **13** weeks, **5** days   Days to due date: **184**

Notes: _____

I'm thirsty in here.
I now drink about
a pint of amniotic
fluid a day.

Today is [/ /]   **13** weeks, **6** days   Days to due date: **183**

Notes: _____

What goes in,
must come out.
Yes, whatever I drink
I urinate back into
the amniotic fluid.

Today is [/ /]   **14** weeks, **0** days   Days to due date: **182**

Notes: _____

I'm moving all over
the place now, but
you may not feel me yet
because I'm so small.

Today is [/ /]   **14** weeks, **1** days   Days to due date: **181**

Notes: _____
_____
_____
_____
_____
_____
_____
_____
_____
_____
_____

Finally, the placenta is fully formed! The placenta nourishes me, gives me oxygen, and disposes my waste.

Today is ___/___/___   **14** weeks, **2** days   Days to due date: **180**

Notes: _____
_____
_____
_____
_____
_____
_____
_____
_____
_____

I'm no giraffe, but my neck is now well defined, and my head rests on my neck instead of my shoulders.

Today is ___/___/___   **14** weeks, **3** days   Days to due date: **179**

Notes: _____
_____
_____
_____
_____
_____
_____
_____

If you could touch my lips, I would suck your finger.

Today is ___/___/___   **14** weeks, **4** days   Days to due date: **178**

Notes: _____

I'm definitely putting on weight. I'm about 2½ ounces (70 grams), which is about as heavy as a hot dog bun.

Today is [/   /   ]   **14** weeks, **5** days   Days to due date: **177**

Notes: _____

Don't be alarmed if you feel jerking sensations, I probably just have the hiccups. They don't make any sound because my trachea is filled with fluid, not air.

Today is [/   /   ]   **14** weeks, **6** days   Days to due date: **176**

Notes: _____

My body is covered with lanugo—a soft, downy hair. I won't need it later, so I'll shed most of it before I'm born.

Today is [/   /   ]   **15** weeks, **0** days   Days to due date: **175**

Notes: _____

During this month, my heart will pump 25 quarts (27.5 liters) of blood a day. By the time I'm born, that amount will increase to 300 quarts per day!

Today is ___ / ___ / ___   15 weeks, 1 days   Days to due date: **174**

Notes: _____

The detailed design of every body part is amazing. All the "instructions" came with the genes you gave me at conception. Thanks, Mom and Dad!

Today is ___ / ___ / ___   15 weeks, 2 days   Days to due date: **173**

Notes: _____

Back off, bacteria! I'm in a completely sterile environment inside my amniotic sac, where you can't get me.

Today is ___ / ___ / ___   15 weeks, 3 days   Days to due date: **172**

Notes: _____

I'm now 6 inches long (15 centimeters) or about as long as a dollar bill. I weigh around 3 ounces (85 grams), which is approximately the weight of a C battery.

Today is / /   **15** weeks, **4** days   Days to due date: **171**

Notes: _____

Soon, I'll have my very own unique fingerprints.

Today is / /   **15** weeks, **5** days   Days to due date: **170**

Notes: _____

Now I'm better proportioned as my body catches up with that big head of mine.

Today is / /   **15** weeks, **6** days   Days to due date: **169**

Notes: _____

Clap for joy! My arms are now long enough for me to hold my hands together.

Today is   /   /   **16** weeks, **0** days   Days to due date: **168**

Notes: _____

My taste buds are more refined. If there's a bitter substance in the amniotic fluid, I'll grimace and stop swallowing the liquid.

Today is   /   /   **16** weeks, **1** days   Days to due date: **167**

Notes: _____

Believe it or not, I can see in here! If you shine a bright light on your belly, I'll gradually move my hands to cover my eyes.

Today is   /   /   **16** weeks, **2** days   Days to due date: **166**

Notes:

Feeling warm? That's because the amniotic fluid is 99.5°F (37.5°C), which is higher than your normal body temperature.

Today is   /   /   **16** weeks, **3** days   Days to due date: **165**

Notes:

I may suck my thumb in here. It helps my coordination and strengthens my jaw and cheek muscles.

Today is   /   /   **16** weeks, **4** days   Days to due date: **164**

Notes:

This has been a week of rapid growth for me. I'm now about 5 ounces (142 grams) or as heavy as a baseball.

Today is   /   /   **16** weeks, **5** days   Days to due date: **163**

Notes: _____
_____
_____
_____

My nostrils used to be wide apart and pointed forward. Now they're moving closer together and pointing downward. Ah, the sweet smell of success!

Today is _____/_____/_____   **16** weeks, **6** days   Days to due date: **162**

Notes: _____
_____
_____
_____

By the time I'm born, I'll display more than 70 different reflex behaviors, such as swallowing, sucking, and clasping my hands. I'm practicing a lot of them now.

Today is _____/_____/_____   **17** weeks, **0** days   Days to due date: **161**

Notes: _____
_____
_____

I can't wiggle and wink them yet, but my eyebrows and eyelashes are growing.

Today is _____/_____/_____   **17** weeks, **1** days   Days to due date: **160**

Notes: _____

My eyes begin to make very slow movements beneath my lids. I can't wait to look around.

Today is ___ / ___ / ___   **17** weeks, **2** days   Days to due date: **159**

Notes: _____

My ears stand out from my head, as they should. Now I have something to hold up my sunglasses when I'm older.

Today is ___ / ___ / ___   **17** weeks, **3** days   Days to due date: **158**

Notes: _____

Vernix caseosa covers my skin. It's a waxy coating that protects my wrinkly skin from the amniotic fluid. Just picture how you'd look after nine months in a bathtub!

Today is ___ / ___ / ___   **17** weeks, **4** days   Days to due date: **157**

Notes: _____
_____
_____
_____

I'm now approximately as long as a dinner fork—about 8 inches (20 centimeters). I weigh 7 ounces (198 grams). That's as heavy as three extra large eggs.
_____
_____
_____
_____
_____
_____

Today is ___ / ___ / ___   **17** weeks, **5** days   Days to due date: **156**

Notes: _____
_____
_____
_____

Call the nail salon—my nail beds now have hard fingernails and toenails that will continue to grow.
_____
_____
_____
_____
_____

Today is ___ / ___ / ___   **17** weeks, **6** days   Days to due date: **155**

Notes: _____
_____
_____
_____

My toes will take longer to develop than my fingers, but don't worry—they'll catch up.
_____
_____
_____
_____
_____

Today is ___ / ___ / ___   **18** weeks, **0** days   Days to due date: **154**

Notes: _____

What's that ruckus? If you make a loud sound, I may raise my hands and cover my ears.

Today is ___/___/___   **18** weeks, **1** days   Days to due date: **153**

Notes: _____

I thought I tasted salt! The amniotic fluid has the salinity of the primeval sea.

Today is ___/___/___   **18** weeks, **2** days   Days to due date: **152**

Notes: _____

My foot is just an inch long now. I don't think they make shoes in my size.

Today is ___/___/___   **18** weeks, **3** days   Days to due date: **151**

COUNTDOWN TO MY BIRTH

Notes: _____

Please don't disturb me. I sleep as much as a newborn—about 18 hours a day!

Today is ___/___/___   **18** weeks, **4** days   Days to due date: **150**

Notes: _____

My "house" cleans itself regularly. The amniotic fluid completely regenerates itself every 3–4 hours.

Today is ___/___/___   **18** weeks, **5** days   Days to due date: **149**

Notes: _____

I love hearing blood flow through your veins and your heart swoosh—it's so comforting.

Today is ___/___/___   **18** weeks, **6** days   Days to due date: **148**

Notes: _____

My senses are coming alive. My sense of taste is now formed, and I can distinguish between bitter and sweet.

Today is ____ / ____ / ____   **19** weeks, **0** days   Days to due date: **147**

Notes: _____

If I'm a girl, I already have approximately 6 million eggs in my ovaries. By the time I'm born, they'll dwindle to around 1 million.

Today is ____ / ____ / ____   **19** weeks, **1** days   Days to due date: **146**

Notes: _____

I'm moving, punching, kicking, and twisting about 200 times a day. That's what I call a workout!

Today is ____ / ____ / ____   **19** weeks, **2** days   Days to due date: **145**

Notes: _____

My legs are getting longer and are now proportionate to the rest of my body. Some day I'll be able to run!

Today is [/   /   ]   **19** weeks, **3** days   Days to due date: **144**

Notes: _____

I'm approximately 9 inches (24 centimeters) long, and I weigh around 10 ounces (283 grams). So, I'm as long as a banana and as heavy as a large orange.

Today is [/   /   ]   **19** weeks, **4** days   Days to due date: **143**

Notes: _____

I'll need a pretty thick skin to make it out there. My skin is thickening to cover and protect my insides.

Today is [/   /   ]   **19** weeks, **5** days   Days to due date: **142**

Notes:

Don't be surprised if you feel me doing somersaults for about two more months—I'm just having fun!

Today is ___ / ___ / ___   **19** weeks, **6** days   Days to due date: **141**

Notes:

Congratulations! We made it to the halfway mark!

Today is ___ / ___ / ___   **20** weeks, **0** days   Days to due date: **140**

Notes:

The fluid in my amniotic sac is increasing, and there's about a pint at this point. That's about how much water is in a large drinking glass.

Today is ___ / ___ / ___   **20** weeks, **1** days   Days to due date: **139**

Notes: _____

I need a lot of nourishment and oxygen in here. Thankfully, you're taking good care of me, Mom. I've noticed your blood volume has increased 30–50 percent to accommodate my needs.

Today is ___ / ___ / ___   **20** weeks, **2** days   Days to due date: **138**

Notes: _____

I'm hungry even if you're not, so try not to skip meals!

Today is ___ / ___ / ___   **20** weeks, **3** days   Days to due date: **137**

Notes: _____

My sense of smell is now complete. I'll smell all sorts of new things when I'm out of here!

Today is ___ / ___ / ___   **20** weeks, **4** days   Days to due date: **136**

Notes: _____

B elieve it or not, I still
weigh less than a pound.
I'm just around 13 ounces
(369 grams). Only 1 percent
of my body weight is fat.

Today is [/ /]   **20** weeks, **5** days   Days to due date: **135**

Notes: _____

M y eyebrows and eyelids
are now fully developed,
but I can't look around yet
because my lids are fused shut
for another month or so.

Today is [/ /]   **20** weeks, **6** days   Days to due date: **134**

Notes: _____

F inally, my fingernails
have grown long enough
to cover my fingertips.

Today is [/ /]   **21** weeks, **0** days   Days to due date: **133**

I can tell when you're sleeping on your left side—that helps your blood flow freely to me.

Notes:

Today is ___ / ___ / ___   **21** weeks, **1** days   Days to due date: **132**

My heart is getting stronger and stronger each day. You can probably hear it with just a stethoscope—you don't need a Doppler ultrasound anymore.

Notes:

Today is ___ / ___ / ___   **21** weeks, **2** days   Days to due date: **131**

No more shark tales—much of my cartilage skeleton has hardened into bone.

Notes:

Today is ___ / ___ / ___   **21** weeks, **3** days   Days to due date: **130**

COUNTDOWN TO MY BIRTH

Notes:

L isten to this: The three bones in my middle ear—the hammer, anvil, and stirrup—are beginning to harden.

Today is   /   /   **21** weeks, **4** days   Days to due date: **129**

Notes:

I 'm almost 11 inches (28 centimeters) long and weigh about 15 ounces (425 grams). That's the length and weight of a football, Dad!

Today is   /   /   **21** weeks, **5** days   Days to due date: **128**

Notes:

I have no trouble finding and playing with my nose, hands, or umbilical cord. It keeps me amused!

Today is   /   /   **21** weeks, **6** days   Days to due date: **127**

Notes: _____

B rown fat, which keeps
me warm at birth, is
developing under my skin.
In this case, lots of fat is good!

Today is ___/___/___   **22** weeks, **0** days   Days to due date: **126**

Notes: _____

I love to move to the beat
of music! Can you feel
me dancing?

Today is ___/___/___   **22** weeks, **1** days   Days to due date: **125**

Notes: _____

A ll my body parts have
caught up to one another,
and now I'm proportioned like
a skinny newborn.

Today is ___/___/___   **22** weeks, **2** days   Days to due date: **124**

Notes:

My eyes are developed, but my irises still don't have pigment. I wonder what color they'll be!

Today is ___/___/___   **22** weeks, **3** days   Days to due date: **123**

Notes:

My eyes can move rapidly now. Too bad my eyelids won't open yet!

Today is ___/___/___   **22** weeks, **4** days   Days to due date: **122**

Notes:

Go into the fridge and pick up a box of butter (four sticks). This is how heavy I am—about a pound (454 grams).

Today is ___/___/___   **22** weeks, **5** days   Days to due date: **121**

Notes: _____
_____
_____
_____
_____
_____
_____
_____
_____
_____

Although it's getting thicker, my skin is still a little transparent. You can see my veins and bones through it. I look a bit like a road map.

Today is ____/____/____   **22** weeks, **6** days   Days to due date: **120**

Notes: _____
_____
_____
_____
_____
_____
_____
_____
_____
_____

Make sure Daddy talks to me whenever he can, too. That way, I'll recognize both of your voices after I'm born.

Today is ____/____/____   **23** weeks, **0** days   Days to due date: **119**

Notes: _____
_____
_____
_____
_____
_____
_____
_____
_____
_____

I love listening to all types of music and can tell the differences among them. Play some classical for me, please. I especially like that!

Today is ____/____/____   **23** weeks, **1** days   Days to due date: **118**

Notes: _____
_____
_____
_____

Take a deep breath: I'm now working on the blood vessels in my lungs to prepare for breathing.

_____
_____
_____
_____
_____
_____

Today is [/   /   ]   **23** weeks, **2** days   Days to due date: **117**

Notes: _____
_____
_____
_____

My skin is growing faster than the tissue beneath it, which is why I look all wrinkly.

_____
_____
_____
_____
_____

Today is [/   /   ]   **23** weeks, **3** days   Days to due date: **116**

Notes: _____
_____
_____
_____

My hearing is perfectly developed, so feel free to read, talk, or sing to me. You don't need special equipment—I can hear you just fine.

_____
_____
_____
_____
_____

Today is [/   /   ]   **23** weeks, **4** days   Days to due date: **115**

Notes: _____

I'm now about 11.8 inches (30 centimeters) long, and I weigh about 1 pound 5 ounces (595 grams). Hey, Dad—I'm as heavy as an official NBA basketball!

Today is ___/___/___ **23** weeks, **5** days Days to due date: **114**

Notes: _____

I'm kicking as hard as I can. If you haven't felt me move yet, give it a few more days—I'm still pretty small.

Today is ___/___/___ **23** weeks, **6** days Days to due date: **113**

Notes: _____

If you could hold my little hands and feet, you'd see that my fingerprints and toe prints are now visible. I won't visit a fortuneteller any time soon, but I also have lines on my palms.

Today is ___/___/___ **24** weeks, **0** days Days to due date: **112**

Notes: _____

Inside my lungs, amazing things are happening. My air sacs are forming rapidly and will continue to form until I'm eight years old.

Today is ____ / ____ / ____   **24** weeks, **1** days   Days to due date: **111**

Notes: _____

Surfactant is developing in my lungs. This substance prevents the air sacs from sticking together, which is a very important part of breathing after I'm born. It's like a lube job for my lungs!

Today is ____ / ____ / ____   **24** weeks, **2** days   Days to due date: **110**

Notes: _____

Boo! I just learned the blink-startle reflex. I have many more reflexes to learn before I'm born.

Today is ____ / ____ / ____   **24** weeks, **3** days   Days to due date: **109**

Notes: _____
_____
_____
_____
_____
_____
_____
_____
_____
_____
_____

Is it hot in here?
My sweat glands
begin to form in
my skin.

Today is _____ / _____ / _____   **24** weeks, **4** days   Days to due date: **108**

Notes: _____
_____
_____
_____
_____
_____
_____
_____
_____
_____
_____

I'm getting bigger. I'm
now about 1 pound 9 ounces
(709 grams), which is roughly
as heavy as a mug of cocoa.

Today is _____ / _____ / _____   **24** weeks, **5** days   Days to due date: **107**

Notes: _____
_____
_____
_____
_____
_____
_____
_____
_____
_____
_____

I'm practicing my breathing
movements, but I don't take
any air into my lungs yet.

Today is _____ / _____ / _____   **24** weeks, **6** days   Days to due date: **106**

COUNTDOWN TO MY BIRTH

A day-by-day account from your baby's point of view

Notes: _____

I already favor one of my hands. Will I be a lefty or a righty?

Today is ___/___/___   **25** weeks, **0** days   Days to due date: **105**

Notes: _____

I'm a creature of habit—even in here—and my movements have fallen into a routine.

Today is ___/___/___   **25** weeks, **1** days   Days to due date: **104**

Notes: _____

As more fat is deposited and my muscles develop, my skin will eventually smooth out. I won't look like such a prune!

Today is ___/___/___   **25** weeks, **2** days   Days to due date: **103**

Notes: _____

My spine consists of 33 rings, 150 joints, and 1,000 ligaments. You have only 24 rings, 116 joints, and many fewer than 1,000 ligaments. Why is that? (I have no idea!)

Today is ___/___/___   **25** weeks, **3** days   Days to due date: **102**

Notes: _____

My capillaries (very small blood vessels) are developing, giving me a reddish glow.

Today is ___/___/___   **25** weeks, **4** days   Days to due date: **101**

Notes: _____

Look at a ruler—I'm about 12–13 inches (30–33 centimeters) now. I weigh approximately 1 pound 12 ounces (794 grams).

Today is ___/___/___   **25** weeks, **5** days   Days to due date: **100**

Notes: _____
_____
_____
_____
_____
_____
_____
_____
_____
_____
_____

I actually dream
when I sleep.
Sweet dreams, Mom!

Today is ___/___/___   **25** weeks, **6** days   Days to due date: **99**

Notes: _____
_____
_____
_____
_____
_____
_____
_____
_____
_____
_____

I'm developing a very
strong grip—test it
out after I'm born!

Today is ___/___/___   **26** weeks, **0** days   Days to due date: **98**

Notes: _____
_____
_____
_____
_____
_____
_____
_____
_____
_____

I'll gain about a pound this
month. Keep "feeding" me
yummy, healthful foods.

Today is ___/___/___   **26** weeks, **1** days   Days to due date: **97**

Notes: _____

It's taken time for my reproductive organs to develop. At the beginning, I didn't look like a girl or a boy, but my genitals continue to be better formed. Thanks, Dad, for giving me the gene to make me what I am!

Today is ___ / ___ / ___   26 weeks, 2 days   Days to due date: **96**

Notes: _____

When I'm born, I'll have 500,000 hair follicles on my skin—100,000 of them will be on my head. That's a lot!

Today is ___ / ___ / ___   26 weeks, 3 days   Days to due date: **95**

Notes: _____

Race you! Blood is flowing through my umbilical cord at 4 miles per hour. A roundtrip through the cord and through my body takes only 30 seconds.

Today is ___ / ___ / ___   26 weeks, 4 days   Days to due date: **94**

Notes:

In the last four weeks, my weight has doubled. I now weigh around 2 pounds (908 grams).

Today is   /   /   **26** weeks, **5** days   Days to due date: **93**

Notes:

My sucking reflex is now well developed in preparation for feeding, preferably from the breast. If you nurse me, even for a short time, I'll receive numerous antibodies and other benefits. I was made to breastfeed!

Today is   /   /   **26** weeks, **6** days   Days to due date: **92**

Notes:

I need more room in here, so I have to push your uterus up into your rib cage. I'm sorry if that causes you to be short of breath and have indigestion!

Today is   /   /   **27** weeks, **0** days   Days to due date: **91**

Notes: _____

Open sesame! My vision is the last sense to develop, but now my eyes can finally open after being fused shut. As I look around, I see shadows.

Today is ___/___/___   27 weeks, **1** days   Days to due date: **90**

Notes: _____

My brain is developing hundreds of billions of nerve cells. Although it won't develop new cells after birth, it will make connections between them every time I learn!

Today is ___/___/___   27 weeks, **2** days   Days to due date: **89**

Notes: _____

Don't worry, your belly can get only so big. I'm now in the fetal position with my legs tucked up to make the most of the space.

Today is ___/___/___   27 weeks, **3** days   Days to due date: **88**

Notes:

The sound of your voice calms and soothes me. When I hear it, my heart rate slows.

Today is ____ / ____ / ____   **27** weeks, **4** days   Days to due date: **87**

Notes:

I weigh 2 pounds 4 ounces (1 kilogram)—slightly less than a jar of spaghetti sauce. I'm also 13.8 inches (35 centimeters) long.

Today is ____ / ____ / ____   **27** weeks, **5** days   Days to due date: **86**

Notes:

The placenta has been very important, but as my body becomes more self-sufficient, I use the placenta less and less.

Today is ____ / ____ / ____   **27** weeks, **6** days   Days to due date: **85**

Notes: _____

We're in the homestretch! The third trimester is beginning!

Today is ___/___/___   **28** weeks, **0** days   Days to due date: **84**

Notes: _____

Think happy thoughts! Your emotions release hormones that cross the placenta, and I feel those emotions.

Today is ___/___/___   **28** weeks, **1** days   Days to due date: **83**

Notes: _____

I'm getting a little plumper as my body stores some fat. I now have 2–3 percent body fat. (A healthy woman has 25–31 percent; a healthy man has 18–25 percent.)

Today is ___/___/___   **28** weeks, **2** days   Days to due date: **82**

Notes:

I'm not sad, but I may cry at times.

Today is ___ / ___ / ___   **28** weeks, **3** days   Days to due date: **81**

Notes:

My body is getting better at regulating my temperature, but even after I'm born, I'll need blankets and your warm skin to keep me from getting cold.

Today is ___ / ___ / ___   **28** weeks, **4** days   Days to due date: **80**

Notes:

I now weigh around 2 pounds 9 ounces (1.16 kilograms)—about as much as a liter of soda pop.

Today is ___ / ___ / ___   **28** weeks, **5** days   Days to due date: **79**

Notes: _____

I'll be born with 300 bones
in my body. As I grow,
some bones will fuse together,
and I'll end up with 206 bones,
just like you.

Today is ___ / ___ / ___   **28** weeks, **6** days   Days to due date: **78**

Notes: _____

I don't mind if you put up
your feet, take a nap, or
read a book. It'll be good
for both of us!

Today is ___ / ___ / ___   **29** weeks, **0** days   Days to due date: **77**

Notes: _____

My brain is in full swing,
developing its different
sections, and it'll continue to
grow rapidly until I'm about
five years old.

Today is ___ / ___ / ___   **29** weeks, **1** days   Days to due date: **76**

Notes: _____

My body is producing hormones that circulate in my blood, cross the placenta, and stimulate your milk production. I want to make sure you have plenty of food for me when the time comes!

Today is ___ / ___ / ___   **29** weeks, **2** days   Days to due date: **75**

Notes: _____

My bone marrow is now ready to make my red blood cells; before now, my spleen handled the job. It's great teamwork!

Today is ___ / ___ / ___   **29** weeks, **3** days   Days to due date: **74**

Notes: _____

Try playing "Name That Bump" and see if you can find my arms, legs, and head. It's fun!

Today is ___ / ___ / ___   **29** weeks, **4** days   Days to due date: **73**

Notes: _____

Right now, I'm approximately 15 inches (38 centimeters) long—like a bowling pin—and I weigh 2½–3 pounds (1.13–1.36 kilograms).

Today is ___/___/___   **29** weeks, **5** days   Days to due date: **72**

Notes: _____

I've been growing taller, but now it's time to put on some pounds. From now on, my weight gain will exceed my length gain.

Today is ___/___/___   **29** weeks, **6** days   Days to due date: **71**

Notes: _____

Even though I'm surrounded by fluid, I don't drown because I don't depend on my lungs yet for air. I receive all my oxygen through my umbilical cord.

Today is ___/___/___   **30** weeks, **0** days   Days to due date: **70**

Notes: _____

B y now I may have settled into a vertex or head-down position. But I can change position up to the last minute!

Today is ___ / ___ / ___   **30** weeks, **1** days   Days to due date: **69**

Notes: _____

A lthough I have lots of hair follicles, those are just the "holes" where hair will eventually grow. That means I may have a lot of hair on my head now, or I may be fairly bald. Either way is completely normal.

Today is ___ / ___ / ___   **30** weeks, **2** days   Days to due date: **68**

Notes: _____

M y brain is growing so rapidly now, it has to fold over itself and wrinkle up in order to fit inside my skull.

Today is ___ / ___ / ___   **30** weeks, **3** days   Days to due date: **67**

COUNTDOWN TO MY BIRTH
A day-by-day account from your baby's point of view

Notes:

Most of my organs are nearly mature, but my lungs still need to develop before I can enter your world.

Today is   /   /   **30** weeks, **4** days   Days to due date: **66**

Notes:

I'm now about 3 pounds 5 ounces (1.5 kilograms)—about as heavy as a cantaloupe.

Today is   /   /   **30** weeks, **5** days   Days to due date: **65**

Notes:

As I grow inside my cramped quarters, my movements may slow down and become less forceful. No more somersaults for me!

Today is   /   /   **30** weeks, **6** days   Days to due date: **64**

Notes: _____

I'm beginning my final growth spurt. I'll need lots of nutrients to be big and strong. Keep 'em coming.

Today is ___/___/___   **31** weeks, **0** days   Days to due date: **63**

Notes: _____

I'm becoming quite the little human being. I have all five senses, I'm aware of my surroundings, and I'm quite intelligent, if I do say so myself!

Today is ___/___/___   **31** weeks, **1** days   Days to due date: **62**

Notes: _____

As I stretch my legs, don't be surprised if I stick my toes up into your rib cage!

Today is ___/___/___   **31** weeks, **2** days   Days to due date: **61**

Notes: _____

My fingernails have gotten pretty long! Don't be alarmed to find scratches on my face when I'm born. They'll heal in a few days.

Today is ___/___/___   **31** weeks, **3** days   Days to due date: **60**

Notes: _____

I can tell when you're out in the sun or under bright lights. My pupils constrict and dilate to varying light, and I can see dim shapes.

Today is ___/___/___   **31** weeks, **4** days   Days to due date: **59**

Notes: _____

Bang the drum! I'm now about 15.8 inches (40 centimeters), which is as long as a drumstick, and I weigh 3 pounds 11 ounces (1.7 kilograms).

Today is ___/___/___   **31** weeks, **5** days   Days to due date: **58**

Notes: _____

My bones continue to grow and harden. I'll be skipping around before you know it.

Today is ___ / ___ / ___   **31** weeks, **6** days   Days to due date: **57**

Notes: _____

I'm no Rapunzel, but the hair on my head is getting longer.(If I have hair, that is!)

Today is ___ / ___ / ___   **32** weeks, **0** days   Days to due date: **56**

Notes: _____

Over the past week, my rapid brain development has increased my head circumference by another ⅜ inch (9.5 millimeters). Imagine how smart I'm going to be!

Today is ___ / ___ / ___   **32** weeks, **1** days   Days to due date: **55**

Notes: _____

I've accomplished so much, but one thing I'll save until a few weeks after I'm born is the completion of my tear ducts. So for those first few cries, you won't see any tears.

Today is ___/___/___   **32** weeks, **2** days   Days to due date: **54**

Notes: _____

Thanks, Mom! Your antibodies flow through the placenta and help protect me from disease.

Today is ___/___/___   **32** weeks, **3** days   Days to due date: **53**

Notes: _____

I wish I could see what "we" look like right now. Please take a picture of your belly to show me someday when I'm older.

Today is ___/___/___   **32** weeks, **4** days   Days to due date: **52**

Notes: _____

I've now hit the 4-pound mark (1.8 kilograms)! In the next seven weeks, my weight will double.

Today is ___/___/___   32 weeks, 5 days   Days to due date: 51

Notes: _____

My gums are ridged, and it looks like my teeth are ready to come through. I could even be born with a few visible teeth!

Today is ___/___/___   32 weeks, 6 days   Days to due date: 50

Notes: _____

My skin is gradually becoming less red and more pink as I build white fat deposits under my skin. I won't have a lot of white fat, however, so I'll still need brown fat deposits for energy and warmth after I'm born.

Today is ___/___/___   33 weeks, 0 days   Days to due date: 49

I like being called "Baby," but I wonder what you're going to call me after I'm born. Have you been thinking about names yet?

Notes: _____

Today is ___ / ___ / ___   **33** weeks, **1** days   Days to due date: **48**

N eurons and synapses are developing like crazy in my brain! These connections will help me learn everything I need to know.

Notes: _____

Today is ___ / ___ / ___   **33** weeks, **2** days   Days to due date: **47**

R emember when I had only 1 percent body fat 13 weeks ago? Well, I've been growing so much, now I have 8 percent.

Notes: _____

Today is ___ / ___ / ___   **33** weeks, **3** days   Days to due date: **46**

Notes: _____

Even though it's crowded in here, don't worry about my umbilical cord. My cord contains Wharton's jelly, a thick goop to prevent it from knotting or kinking.

Today is [/ /]   **33** weeks, **4** days   Days to due date: **45**

Notes: _____

I've really grown lately. I'm about 17 inches (43 centimeters) long, and I weigh approximately 4 pounds 7 ounces (2 kilograms). That's about as heavy as a half gallon of milk.

Today is [/ /]   **33** weeks, **5** days   Days to due date: **44**

Notes: _____

Due to the lack of pigmentation, my eyes are still a slate color, regardless of my race. My true color won't emerge until several weeks after I'm born. Will I have your eyes or Dad's?

Today is [/ /]   **33** weeks, **6** days   Days to due date: **43**

Countdown to My Birth

Notes: _____

You'll be happy to learn that the circumference of my head equals the circumference of my shoulders. That will make delivery easier for both you and me!

Today is ___ / ___ / ___   **34** weeks, **0** days   Days to due date: **42**

Notes: _____

I told you I was going through a growth spurt! I'll gain about 2 pounds (908 grams) this month and will grow almost 3 inches (7.6 centimeters).

Today is ___ / ___ / ___   **34** weeks, **1** days   Days to due date: **41**

Notes: _____

You take good care of me in here, and I know you'll do the same after I'm born. Your milk is made especially for me, and it'll continually change to suit my needs.

Today is ___ / ___ / ___   **34** weeks, **2** days   Days to due date: **40**

Notes: _____

My head used to be huge compared to the rest of my body, but now it's about one-quarter of my total body size.

Today is ____ / ____ / ____   **34** weeks, **3** days   Days to due date: **39**

Notes: _____

Don't worry—99 percent of babies born at this stage survive with no major problems.

Today is ____ / ____ / ____   **34** weeks, **4** days   Days to due date: **38**

Notes: _____

I'm approximately 18 inches (46 centimeters) long and weigh about 4 pounds 12 ounces (2.15 kilograms). Can you believe how big I'm getting?

Today is ____ / ____ / ____   **35** weeks, **5** days   Days to due date: **37**

COUNTDOWN TO MY BIRTH
A day-by-day account from your baby's point of view

Notes: _____

You've made a wonderful home for me these last few months. Your uterus has expanded 1,000 times its original volume. Even with all that space, I'm sorry if I'm still poking your ribs!

Today is ___/___/___   **34** weeks, **6** days   Days to due date: **36**

Notes: _____

Every day I'm in here, my lungs get more and more developed, making it so much easier for me to breathe later.

Today is ___/___/___   **35** weeks, **0** days   Days to due date: **35**

Notes: _____

My goal is to be about 20 inches (51 centimeters) and 7½ pounds (3.4 kilograms) when I'm born—which is the average size for babies. But of course it's okay if I'm a little smaller or larger.

Today is ___/___/___   **35** weeks, **1** days   Days to due date: **34**

Notes: _____

I draw calcium from your body to help strengthen and build my bones. Drink an extra glass of milk for me!

Today is ___ / ___ / ___   **35** weeks, **2** days   Days to due date: **33**

Notes: _____

I may drop lower in your pelvis. This is called lightening. It makes it easier for you to breathe and eat, but uncomfortable to walk.

Today is ___ / ___ / ___   **35** weeks, **3** days   Days to due date: **32**

Notes: _____

We haven't made it to the due date yet, but I could surprise you at any time by arriving early. Be prepared!

Today is ___ / ___ / ___   **35** weeks, **4** days   Days to due date: **31**

Notes: _____

Now I weigh about 5 pounds 2 ounces (2.3 kilograms). Pick up a bag of flour in the store to feel how heavy I am.

Today is ___ / ___ / ___   **35** weeks, **5** days   Days to due date: **30**

Notes: _____

If I'm not there yet, my main job now is to settle head down in your pelvis in preparation for my birth.

Today is ___ / ___ / ___   **35** weeks, **6** days   Days to due date: **29**

Notes: _____

It's pretty cramped in here, so forgive me if I press on your bladder some more.

Today is ___ / ___ / ___   **36** weeks, **0** days   Days to due date: **28**

Notes: _____

Now is definitely not the time for you to diet! During the final weeks, approximately ½ ounce (14 grams) of fat a day builds under my skin.

Today is ___/___/___   36 weeks, 1 days   Days to due date: 27

Notes: _____

You'll soon need to break out the clippers—my toenails have grown long enough to reach the tips of my toes.

Today is ___/___/___   36 weeks, 2 days   Days to due date: 26

Notes: _____

Have you felt my knee pushing on your stomach? Or is that my elbow?

Today is ___/___/___   36 weeks, 3 days   Days to due date: 25

COUNTDOWN TO MY BIRTH
A day-by-day account from your baby's point of view

Notes: _____

G ood news: If I'm like
85 percent of babies,
I'll be born sometime between
two weeks before and two
weeks after my due date.

Today is ___/___/___   **36** weeks, **4** days   Days to due date: **24**

Notes: _____

B irth will be stressful
for me, too, but I'm
well prepared to cope with
it. I'll secrete more hormones,
especially endorphins, during
birth than any other time in
my life.

Today is ___/___/___   **36** weeks, **5** days   Days to due date: **23**

Notes: _____

W ait till you see the little
dimples on my elbows
and knees—they're so cute!

Today is ___/___/___   **36** weeks, **6** days   Days to due date: **22**

Notes: _____

Most of my vernix
caseosa (waxy coating)
has disappeared, as has the
lanugo (downy coating),
but don't laugh if I still have
a few patches after birth.

Today is ___/___/___   37 weeks, **0** days   Days to due date: **21**

Notes: _____

I'm preparing for my first
poopy diaper by collecting
meconium in my intestines.
Sorry, Mom!

Today is ___/___/___   37 weeks, **1** days   Days to due date: **20**

Notes: _____

My lungs are now mature,
but they'll continue to
develop. I'll demonstrate their
capacity soon. (*Wah!*)

Today is ___/___/___   37 weeks, **2** days   Days to due date: **19**

Notes: _____

My brain was one of the first organs that developed, and it'll be the last finished. The connections will keep arranging more and more until I have literally trillions of them.

Today is ___ / ___ / ___   **37** weeks, **3** days   Days to due date: **18**

Notes: _____

By the time I'm born, my original single cell will have divided and grown into several trillion!

Today is ___ / ___ / ___   **37** weeks, **4** days   Days to due date: **17**

Notes: _____

Unbelievable! I'm approximately 20–21 inches long (51–53 centimeters) and weigh about 6½ pounds (3 kilograms).

Today is ___ / ___ / ___   **37** weeks, **5** days   Days to due date: **16**

Notes: _____

Your contractions won't hurt me, whether they're early Braxton-Hicks contractions or the real ones during labor. They'll just squeeze me tightly like big bear hugs.

Today is ___/___/___   **37** weeks, **6** days   Days to due date: **15**

Notes: _____

Great job, Mom! We're considered "full term" as of today! Full term means two weeks before through two weeks after your due date.

Today is ___/___/___   **38** weeks, **0** days   Days to due date: **14**

Notes: _____

When your water breaks, I'll feel the fluid drain past my body. When that happens, I'll know it's time!

Today is ___/___/___   **38** weeks, **1** days   Days to due date: **13**

Notes: _____

I hope this rate doesn't continue, but my weight has increased 6 billion times since I was a single fertilized egg.

Today is ___/___/___   **38** weeks, **2** days   Days to due date: **12**

Notes: _____

Your blood gives me a final boost of antibodies so I can safely meet the outside world. After birth, I'll receive antibodies from your breastmilk.

Today is ___/___/___   **38** weeks, **3** days   Days to due date: **11**

Notes: _____

I'm putting on more of that special brown fat throughout my body. It'll act like a little furnace and generate heat to keep me warm after birth.

Today is ___/___/___   **38** weeks, **4** days   Days to due date: **10**

Notes: _____

Only 3–4 percent of babies are born on their actual due dates, so don't despair if I'm not right on time. Remember, it's called your "estimated due date" for a reason!

Today is ___/___/___   **38** weeks, **5** days   Days to due date: **9**

Notes: _____

My umbilical cord is approximately 20 inches (50.8 centimeters) long and has no pain receptors. So don't worry about hurting me when Dad (or another person) cuts the cord.

Today is ___/___/___   **38** weeks, **6** days   Days to due date: **8**

Notes: _____

As soon as I'm born, my eyes will focus best 8–12 inches (20–30 centimeters) from an object—the distance between my face and yours when you're feeding me.

Today is ___/___/___   **39** weeks, **0** days   Days to due date: **7**

Notes: _____

My skull is made up of five large, bony plates that are still separated. They'll push together and over one another during my birth. Don't worry—my normal shape will return in a few weeks.

Today is ___/___/___   **39** weeks, **1** days   Days to due date: **6**

Notes: _____

I'm still approximately 20–21 inches (51–53 centimeters) long, but I should weigh about 7½ pounds (3.4 kilograms) by now, which is a little less than a gallon of milk.

Today is ___/___/___   **39** weeks, **2** days   Days to due date: **5**

Notes: _____

You're not considered "overdue" until two weeks past your due date, so you can relax. If I'm your first baby, you may go over your due date by an average of 10 days.

Today is ___/___/___   **39** weeks, **3** days   Days to due date: **4**

Notes: _____

Some days I feel your belly tighten all around me, release, then tighten again. Are you practicing for labor?

Today is ____ / ____ / ____   **39** weeks, **4** days   Days to due date: **3**

Notes: _____

I've been preparing for birth my whole life, and my body is mostly ready to face the outside world. My arms, legs, fingers, and toes are all perfectly formed. I can't wait to stretch them out!

Today is ____ / ____ / ____   **39** weeks, **5** days   Days to due date: **2**

Notes: _____

My stomach, kidneys, digestive tract, and other organs are getting ready for the big day when I eat my first meal "out."

Today is ____ / ____ / ____   **39** weeks, **6** days   Days to due date: **1**

COUNTDOWN TO MY BIRTH
A day-by-day account from your baby's point of view

Notes: _____

CONGRATULATIONS! You made it to your due date. If I haven't arrived yet, it just means I'm working on a few more details, and it should be any day now. I can't wait to meet you!

Today is ___/___/___   **40** weeks, **0** days   Days past due date: **0**

Notes: _____

I'll miss this warm, cozy home! I'm used to tight spaces, so for the first few weeks after birth, I may like being swaddled.

Today is ___/___/___   **40** weeks, **1** days   Days past due date: **1**

Notes: _____

You've been a tremendous help, Mom, but by now my brain has made trillions of connections and is prepared to take control of my body. I'll make more and more of these connections and get smarter and smarter until I'm born!

Today is ___/___/___   **40** weeks, **2** days   Days past due date: **2**

COUNTDOWN TO MY BIRTH
A day-by-day account from your baby's point of view

Remember that old saying, "The baby will come when the baby is ready"? I want to wait for exactly the right moment, so please be patient with me.

Today is ___/___/___   **40** weeks, **3** days   Days past due date: **3**

Breathing will be my biggest triumph once I'm born. I now have enough surfactant to easily inflate my lungs. My lungs will keep developing right up to my birth.

Today is ___/___/___   **40** weeks, **4** days   Days past due date: **4**

Any day now! When it's time, my brain will send a message to my pituitary gland. A chain reaction of chemicals and hormones will jump-start my adrenal glands, which will then send a stress hormone through my umbilical cord to the placenta.

Today is ___/___/___   **40** weeks, **5** days   Days past due date: **5**

But it doesn't end there! Once the placenta receives its signal, it'll produce and release estrogen. This will make your cervix soften and open slightly. Once that happens, we'll both need to release oxytocin to speed up those contractions.

Notes: _____

Today is ___/___/___   **40** weeks, **6** days   Days past due date: **6**

During my delivery I'll face your side through the birth canal, then I'll turn toward your back to let the pointy part of my head go through first. Once I see daylight, I'll turn again toward your side to let my shoulders and body slip through.

Notes: _____

Today is ___/___/___   **41** weeks, **0** days   Days past due date: **7**

I practice my breathing by actually inhaling the amniotic fluid as if it were air. The pushing and tightening during birth will squeeze that amniotic fluid from my lungs. When I cry out for the first time, my air sacs will open to receive the oxygen.

Notes: _____

Today is ___/___/___   **41** weeks, **1** days   Days past due date: **8**

COUNTDOWN TO MY BIRTH
A day-by-day account from your baby's point of view

I've been in a nice, sterile environment for the last nine months, so I'm not used to bacteria. When I arrive, I'll stay healthier if you ask visitors to please wash their hands before holding me.

Notes:

Today is ___/___/___   **41** weeks, **2** days   Days past due date: **9**

Right now, blood bypasses my lungs because I receive all my oxygen through the umbilical cord. Once I take my first breath, these bypasses will close forever, and oxygen-rich blood will thankfully flow into my lungs.

Notes:

Today is ___/___/___   **41** weeks, **3** days   Days past due date: **10**

When my cord is cut, it'll signal the end of my physical connection to you. We're a good team, but soon I'll be my own person. I'll just need your help in other ways!

Notes:

Today is ___/___/___   **41** weeks, **4** days   Days past due date: **11**

Notes: _____

I'm looking forward to the day I can feel your arms around me, but until then, my body is still putting on the finishing touches. Please don't rush me!

Today is _____ / _____ / _____   **41** weeks, **5** days   Days to due date: **12**

Notes: _____

Once I'm born, treasure every moment with me. It's not every day you get to meet a miracle!

Today is _____ / _____ / _____   **41** weeks, **6** days   Days to due date: **13**

Notes:

Notes:

Notes:

Also from Meadowbrook Press

100,000+ Baby Names by Bruce Lansky is the #1 baby name book and the most complete guide for helping you name your baby. It contains more than 100,000 popular and unusual names from around the world, complete with origins, meanings, variations, and famous namesakes. It also includes the most recent list of top 100 names for girls and boys, and over 600 helpful lists of names to consider and avoid.

Pregnancy, Childbirth, and the Newborn by Penny Simkin et al, was created to help expectant mothers make informed decisions throughout their pregnancy. Completely redesigned, this authoritative book has become the "bible" for childbirth educators.

Baby Play & Learn Child-development expert Penny Warner offers 160 ideas for games and activities that provide hours of developmental learning opportunities. It includes bulleted lists of skills baby learns through play, step-by-step instructions for each game and activity, and illustrations that demonstrate how to play many of the games.

First-Year Baby Care, edited by Paula Kelly MD, is one of the leading guides to your baby's first year. It contains complete information on the basics of baby care, including bathing, diapering, medical facts, and feeding your baby. Now recently revised.

Baby & Child Emergency First Aid edited by Mitchell J. Einzig MD and Paula Kelly MD. This user-friendly book is the next best thing to 911, with a quick-reference index, large illustrations, and easy-to-read instructions on handling the most common childhood emergencies.

We offer many more titles written to delight, inform, and entertain. To browse our full selection of titles, visit our web site at:

www.MeadowbrookPress.com

For quantity discounts, please call: 1-800-338-2232

Meadowbrook Press